Eat Healthy, Feel Better, Live Longer
Copyright 2008, Dr. Robert D. Bard, OD, FAAO, ONS

## Table of Contents

# Introduction

Hello, I'm Dr. Bob, the Health Builder. I want to tell you about a Health Builder Program that I've discovered. If you're overweight or unhealthy, or if you have friends or family who are, this is a Health Builder Program to lose weight and regain your health. It's easy to do, but you do have to change your lifestyle. There are some things you have to learn, but they are not hard. You can't fall off this plan. If you go out with family and friends and eat something that is not on the plan just start over the next day—don't feel guilty!

There are many things about losing weight and eating healthy that you're not told. Most of us have been told that if we're fat and overweight it's because we sit around like couch potatoes, and that's not completely true. Following my Health Builder Program will give you ten important and positive results:

- ➡ You'll feel better.

- ➡ You'll look better.

- ➡ You'll look younger.

- ➡ You'll become more physically active; you'll feel more like doing things.

➡ You'll have more endurance, stamina and staying power, enhancing all your physical activities.

➡ You'll live longer with a better quality of life. It's not so much that you need to live to be 100, but *however* long you live, you want a good quality of life. You don't want to rely on multiple medications, be unable to enjoy life—and maybe even be too broke to buy food because you're spending $1,000 or $1,200 a month on drugs.

➡ You'll breathe better. Before this program, my breathing was hard when I bent over, but not afterwards.

➡ You'll have better self esteem; you'll feel good about yourself.

➡ You'll be admired by your family and friends because of what you've done.

➡ And this one is kind of important—you'll have better sex and better sex appeal.

To get into the plan, there are some things you need to know. The reason I'm writing this book is because I don't believe diets work, but you need to know the specifics of eating healthy and losing weight.

So, welcome to Dr. Bob's Health Builder Program. I wrote this book is because I have had health problems, and I've proven that you can solve them. Some people have tried my recommendations, lost weight and became healthier. It's not that difficult.

Whenever you talk about weight loss and health, some people whine and cry that they can't lose weight. The truth is that a lot of people don't want to lose weight. For those people, there's nothing I can do; there's nothing anybody can do. If you don't care, you don't care.

But for those who do care, this system will help you look better, feel better and improve other aspects of your life.

My weight problem was at least partly caused by eating the wrong things. Fortunately, I found out what *not* to do, and I'm going to share that with you. I also had a health problem, which required using toxic chemicals. One of the results of using those chemicals was that I blew up like the Pillsbury Doughboy. I couldn't get rid of it. My knees hurt and my ankles hurt. It was hard to walk and it was certainly uncomfortable.

Today, I'm a whole lot better. And you can be *too*!

# Should you watch calories?

One of the topics that always comes up about eating healthy and losing weight—and in fact my mother told me recently that I was wrong about my answer—is whether to watch calories.

The answer is absolutely no! If you watch calories, you're setting yourself up to fail. If there's anything you don't want to do it is count calories. But, if you do what I'm suggesting, not only will you be better but you'll get to the point where you don't have the urge to eat all those calories. At some point, it becomes moot because it's just not important. You don't need to count calories. While this is true, there are some exceptions. Avoiding toxic foods and chemicals and cutting "white" foods will take care of the calories, but at some point your body will go into starvation mode (it thinks you are not eating enough), and you will have to count calories and carbs to get out of this mode.

You'll also find there is a lot of emphasis on body measurements. Body measurements are advocated by a lot of people, particularly gyms where you work out. A lot of them tout the BMI, the Body Mass Index. The truth is that it's unimportant. You know if you're overweight. You don't need somebody to say, "Here are the numbers."

Don't worry about it. It makes you frustrated and you don't need that.

## Will doctors and dieticians like your diet, Dr. Bob?

The answer to that is probably not. First of all, the last people you want to get advice from about nutrition are doctors and dieticians. If you don't believe me, go to some institution like a school lunch program which has been set up by dieticians. If you look at the quality of the food, you'll know doggone well they don't know anything about nutrition, because there probably isn't any food in the world worse to give our kids than what's given out by the school lunch program.

With doctors, their nutrition training probably consists of a couple of hours one day out of their entire medical training. Then, they're supposed to be experts on nutrition.

One of the things that bugs the heck out of me is these people who say, "Oh, it's easy to eat nutritious food. Just go to the store and buy fresh fruits and vegetables, and buy the good stuff and not the processed stuff, and you'll be fine."

Well, the problem is they know nothing about nutrition, and if they did, they would tell you that the fruits and vegetables in your grocery store have no trace minerals. The vitamins are very poor and they also have herbicides and pesticides because the farming community hides that from you. So, there is nothing very nutritious about it.

But there are solutions to this and that's the one thing I want you to understand. This isn't a negative program. I'm going to give you things that are positive. If you don't feel like doing all of it now, then don't. But start instituting things I do and say, and you'll get the same results that I did. To give you an idea, I just ordered a pair of pants two weeks ago that are a size 40, and I was wearing a size 50 when I started this program!

Some people will tell you that you have to have a score card, and that's why they like counting calories. But my solution was to not weigh myself. You get on the scale in the morning and you didn't lose any weight, so you get frustrated. You say, "Oh heck, I'll just eat what I want to." I haven't been on the scales more than a few times. I know I've lost about 70 pounds because I know what I weighed before. But the point is you don't want to set yourself up for failure.

My marker is what has happened to my clothing. My shirts are not as tight. My buttons on my shirt aren't tight. That was one of the first things that happened. It was really easy to lose the first 30 or 40 pounds. The rest of it has taken longer, but nonetheless, that first part came off pretty easily in the first four months.

The belt I bought about two and a half years ago fit perfectly then. Now it's about 12 inches too long—maybe 14. I have markers. It's what I do and what I look like. You can tell the difference this program makes without all the things some people think you need to do in terms of measurements. Feeling better is the most important marker.

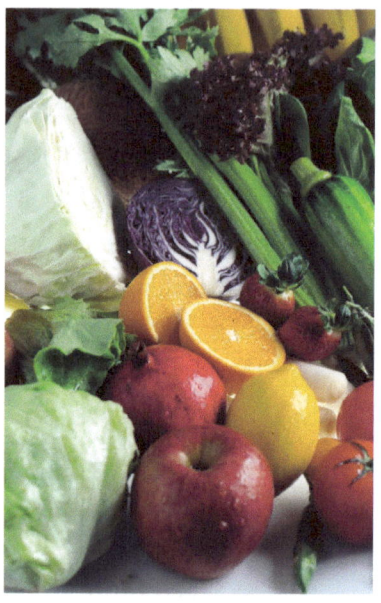

One of the things that we've all seen on television news is that we're a bunch of couch potatoes. We're lazy. We don't work out. We don't do this, we don't do that. The truth is most people are overweight and they don't know why. Now, if they don't care, then there's nothing we can do about it. But, for those who do care, I'm going to instruct you, show you, teach you—whatever word you want to use. I'm going to show you things that you can do to overcome old habits and learn why you gained weight in the first place.

# Do you eat fresh fruits and vegetables?

Absolutely! In fact, one of the things I do every morning is grind up fresh fruits and vegetables in a special, heavy duty blender and make a smoothie. I don't use soy protein. Soy protein is a terrible product, and I'll tell you why later. I don't use sugar or milk. I'll discuss milk later and why you shouldn't drink regular milk.

All I do is put in fresh fruits and vegetables. I use juices sometimes, but I prefer using filtered water. Water is a very important ingredient and I will go over what you should do to get better quality water.

# What about the Food Pyramid?

One of the things we've all seen promoted (in fact they've been running this advertisement on TV) is the Food Pyramid. I want to tell you, the Food Pyramid is not there to help you be healthy. It's there for companies that make processed foods, grains and particularly cereals. It's there to try to convince you to buy more of their junk food. The things on the Food Pyramid for the most part, the ones they advocate the most, are the biggest bunch of junk—things you shouldn't be eating.

I'm going to take each one of these topics, define it, and explain it more thoroughly as we go along.

## Is this a "no carb" diet?

No, it's not. I believe in carbs, but I believe in the right carbs. The carbohydrates I use come from fruits and vegetables. The carbohydrates I don't eat are grains. Why do we put cows in a feed lot? We put them in to get fat. We make them fat by feeding them grain.

Grains make them sick, so they have to be given antibiotics to keep them from becoming infectious. The grain also causes an acid stomach condition, which then causes super e-coli. If people accidentally get e-coli in a hamburger, it can sometimes be deadly.

So, if grain is unhealthy for cows, do you suppose maybe it's unhealthy for people? If you think about it, as grains have been pushed on us, and as we've been advised to cut back fats and meat, guess what? The population began to get bigger and bigger. Grains are one of the biggest reasons that people gain weight and develop disease. Most of them have absolutely no nutrition whatsoever.

# I don't eat white bread, but I eat whole wheat. Is that okay?

First of all, white anything has no nutrition in it. They take wheat, strip the nutrition off, make it white and add chemical vitamins and minerals. Then they want you to believe they fortified it and made it healthful, and that's not true. They haven't made it healthful at all. In fact, they've destroyed everything. The truth is, white bread is terrible, and wheat bread, if you read the label, is the same as white. They just dye it brown and give it a little different taste with chemicals.

Did you know they (industrial food manufactures) put over 3,000 chemicals in food to try to fool your taste buds? It's very easy for them to do. They can trick you, and use almost no real foods. It's amazing what they do with chemicals. It kind of seems to me, and it may be oversimplified, that if God wanted us to have all these chemicals in our bodies, He would have given them to us 3,000 or 4,000 years ago. Since this has just occurred since 1950, I think there's something wrong with our food.

# Cereal for breakfast

One of the things the government promises, or claims, is that the average child can get his or her nutrition in the morning from cereal. If you watch the commercials, that's got to be the greatest thing since sliced bread. But, the truth is. sliced bread isn't healthy, so cereal isn't either. I'm going to give you an example of what that's like. For years, cereal companies have been stripping away all the minerals and vitamins, using white flour. Lately, you've seen the new commercials that tell you they use whole grains and, therefore, it's healthier. They still take the whole grains, make it into "slurry" and extrude it with high pressure and temperature, which reduces it to zero nutrition.

What is extrusion? When manufacturing food, they force it through an opening at high pressure and high temperature. It comes out as a flake, an O, a star or a shredded whatever. The fact is, with the high pressure and high temperature they destroy every bit of vitamins, minerals and nutrition. In fact, the nutrition is absolutely zero.

Even if you go to the health food store and buy corn flakes, you still have zero nutrition because it went through the extrusion process. Even the artificial vitamins the company pumped back into the cereal are destroyed by the process. The only thing that survives is carbohydrates, and the sugar it has in it.

There was a study done a number of years ago. It was done for fun. Honest to goodness, it was done for *fun*. They had 18 rats left over at a university in the North Central part of the U.S. They took the 18 rats and divided them into three groups. Six rats got rat food,

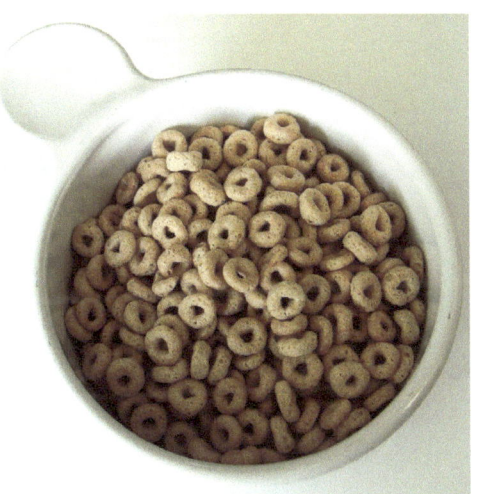

vitamins, minerals and water, and they were watched. The second group got corn flakes, vitamins, minerals and water, and they were watched.

The third group was given the cardboard box that the corn flakes had come in, along with vitamins, minerals and water, and they were watched.

After a period of weeks, the first group to die was the rats that were fed the cereal—in other words, the corn flakes. There was so little nutrition that even the vitamins and minerals that were put in the water could not fortify the rats to live very long. The second group that died was the rats that ate the box. Now, there were six eating the cereal and six eating the box. The day the sixth one from the cereal group died was the day the first one from the box group died.

So, the fact is that the ones that ate the box were healthier. The truth is the cereal box had more nutrition in it than the cereal *in* the box. That's not a pleasant thought, and not a good way to send your child off to school.

## Milk for calcium

One of the things I promised to talk about was milk. We've seen commercials saying that if you drink milk you put calcium in your bones. The research on this is far out of whack. There is no such thing. Milk in the grocery stores is not really milk—it's a white liquid. If you could take the cow that produced the milk and then give that same milk in a bottle back to her, the cow wouldn't recognize it.

Milk processors take the milk, put it in large containers, separate it and then put it back piece by piece. They particularly like to remove the fats. The idea is that fats cause you to be fat and raise your cholesterol. They love to take the fats out of the milk because it removes all the nutrition. At the same time, they get to sell the fats because they go to ice cream and stuff, so they make a lot more money than if they just sold it as whole milk.

Another factor is that there are companies out there that make Genetically Engineered Hormones and give it to cows. When they give these hormones to a cow she

doesn't have to stop being milked for a period of a couple of months—she doesn't need to be bred to have babies. They just keep making her pump out milk. The truth is, dairy cows are one of the most abused animals in the food cycle that we have today. They stand around in cow manure up to their ankles. The farmers wash it down to

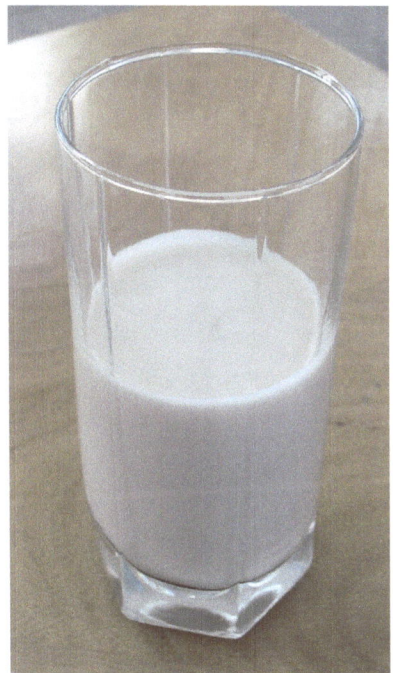

create pollution and that's all they do in the name of cleanliness. The cows are inbred to the point that they can't walk right, and have all kinds of genetic problems.

But, nonetheless, when they give the cows the genetically engineered hormones, this creates white cells. The more hormones they give, the more the white cells go up. This is not a pleasant topic, but when you think of white cells, what is that? Well, it's bacteria. If you really think about what it is, it has to do with pus. The fact is there is a certain amount of pus that is allowed in the milk every day all across the country. Each state is different, but what they do to get rid of that bacterial infectious process is just to heat the milk a lot hotter and destroy more of the nutrition that's in it.

By the time you buy milk in the store, there is absolutely no nutrition left whatsoever. If you like milk, I strongly suggest that you buy organic milk. There are two companies: one is called Horizon and the other is Organic Valley. I buy both because sometimes I don't have a choice. I prefer to buy Organic Valley because it's a co-op of small farmers just trying to make a living by producing a better quality product. Horizon's product is fine, too, but the cows are still fed in confinement, even though they are given feed that is not genetically engineered. Because they are still in confinement, it's not healthy. People that are lactose intolerant are that way because of pasteurization. High heat kills the bacteria but leaves the toxins in the milk.

You'd be much better off to buy non-homogenized, non-pasteurized milk. Now, you're going to say, "Oh, we've been told for years that we need pasteurized milk because otherwise we get diseases!" Percentage–wise, there are more people dying from processed milk than there are from raw milk. Well, the reason you get diseases is because companies are so sloppy in handling fresh milk and the cows are so filthy. They stand around in manure. When the cows are treated properly, not abused, and not put into these dirty waste cycles (or whatever you want to call them), they can produce healthy milk. In fact, there's an organization that's promoting this all over the United States and they're becoming quite successful with it. It is the Westin A. Price Foundation (www.westonaprice.org). Also, avoid ultra-pasteurized milk. The temperature is raised above 225 degrees and destroys all nutrients. It will keep for one month without refrigeration.

## Supplements from the store

Sure, you can simply go to the store and buy supplements, and we all *need* supplements. But supplements in grocery stores are poor quality. I'm not picking on any grocery store. They're in the business of selling food. They're in the business of making money, not selling good health, so why do you think they put pharmacies in food stores? They sell poor, unhealthy food that makes you ill, so you need convenient access to drugs from docs that don't know how to tell you to eat healthy.

The bottom line is that these stores just buy from suppliers, and the suppliers stick them with whatever they have. There are very few benefits from the ones you find on the shelves. In fact, some of the most common ones, nationally known brands, are referred to as "bedpan pellets" because they're not even digested enough to take the name off the pills.

Another example of a mineral that is not good is calcium citrate. It is supposed to replace the calcium in your bones. The problem is that it's the metallic form. The body after the age of 35 will only absorb at the most 7% and probably closer to 4% or 5%. So, the fact is, if you take a supplement to try to replace calcium in your bones, you're going to find out 10 or 15 years later that you're bent over with a hump on your back from the lack of calcium. You end up with osteoporosis—exactly what you were trying to prevent.

## Juice: why is that bad?

There's always the thought that juices are good. We see them advertised. We see orange juice, apple juice and grape juice. But in reality juices are absolutely horrible. Now, I'm not saying the fruit. Remember, I eat fruits and vegetables. The fruit isn't bad because when you consume the fruit you get the juice, but you also get the fiber. You get the solids, you get the trace minerals—you get everything. But when it's juice, processors have strained everything out of it. There is nothing left but carbs. A 12 oz container of juice has 8 teaspoons of sugar. On top of that, they pasteurize it. They've made this into a law so farmers can't compete with corporations. They've tried to destroy artisan producers—the farmers and the people who used to make a good product and would sell it locally. These large corporations have arranged it through the government so that everything has to be pasteurized. One product that I used to love is apple cider, but you cannot buy it in the United States unless it's been pasteurized. I refuse to buy products like that.

So, what are you giving kids when you give them juice? You're giving nothing but carbs, and guess what? If you don't burn carb calories, you store them as fat. That's another reason that children are overweight. Also, the one I really "like" (and I'm being sarcastic) is orange juice. They try to tell you it's pure and it does this and it does that. Again, with the pasteurization, they destroy a lot of the good ingredients. The other thing is, to keep it from settling out, they mix it with a soy lecithin made from soy beans. You can't even drink orange juice without getting soy beans.

We're going to get into soy beans as we go along, but soy beans are one of the unhealthiest foods you can eat. I know the Japanese and the Chinese have eaten tofu for centuries, but they didn't have genetically engineered soy beans. They didn't have soy lecithin, proteins and all of this other stuff thrown into everything imaginable. Soy is fermented in Asia, not consumed as soy.

Another thing that I advocate very heavily is you must read labels! You have to read labels on everything. My philosophy is if you can't read it, you can't spell it or you can't pronounce it, why would you want to put it between your teeth? I want to discuss soy beans and genetically engineered foods, but in the meantime, grow your own foods or buy as much as you can from local people.

Buy oranges and other fruits and veggies. Wash off the chemicals. The fertilizers and the pesticides are on the outside of that orange—you can count on it. Apples are the same way. So you want to clean them and clean them very well. Then take the orange and make orange juice. At that point, you have the pulp left. It's great; it's a good product. But what you get coming through commercially that is man-made is not good. In fact, isn't it interesting that we assume that man can improve on what God made? We need God and his assistance, but we don't need these other products that bypass Him and His good thinking.

# Artificial sweeteners

MANY people use artificial sweeteners. This topic deserves some explaining. The bad part about artificial sweeteners is what they do to the body. They are unnatural chemicals that you should not be putting into your body. There are three sweeteners: Aspartame, Splenda® and Sweet'N Low®. I don't Sweet'N Low comes from a coal tar derivative. Nothing nutritious comes from coal tar derivatives.

Another artificial sweetener is Splenda. The problem with Splenda is we don't really know a lot about it, but we do know it's not natural. The manufacturer starts off with sugar and makes a chlorinated hydrocarbon out of it (this is related to DDT, another chlorinated hydrocarbon). There are all kinds of things on the Internet about why this causes problems. I had a personal friend who ended up very, very ill from this— boils under her breasts and arms—and extreme fatigue, plus a friend that got horrible headaches after a small amount of Splenda. As I said, it's still new enough that we don't know all its side effects, but we do know it was a pesticide before it became a sweetener.

The third one is Aspartame, known by the trade name Equal®; it's the blue stuff. It's in diet drinks and about 6,000 other food products. People think that by using non-caloric sweeteners that they're going to save calories. What they don't know is those same chemicals actually cause them to gain weight. From the Aspartame standpoint, it's called paradoxical weight gain. That's not a good explanation, but sometimes we don't understand how a reaction works. Dr. H. R. Roberts, MD, wrote a good book in the late 1980s on Aspartame and all of its many toxic effects. There is also a new book by Dr Joseph Mercola: *Sweet Deception*.

## Excitotoxins

Aspartame is considered an excitotoxin. It's an amino acid that is genetically engineered and it's very toxic to the body. There is another excitotoxin we've all heard about called MSG, monosodium glutamate. We've always heard that it comes in Chinese food. The truth is that almost all prepared foods (95%) today have MSG in them. Aspartame, hydrolyzed vegetable protein and MSG are excitotoxins. They come from different sources, but they're basically the same kind of product. MSG was a chemical manufactured by the Japanese many years ago. If you put it in foods, it tricks your taste buds into thinking you really taste something good when it's nothing more than chemicals and poor food.

To give an example, if you go to a restaurant where they have au jus, the juice that comes with steak or possibly a roast beef sandwich, you would probably say, "That looks pretty good and has a good taste." The truth of it is, an animal never got close to that stuff. It doesn't have anything to do with the drippings from cooking beef. It is nothing but pure, unadulterated toxic chemicals.

Hydrolyzed vegetable/soy protein is produced by boiling rotten veggies in sulfuric acid until it is mush, neutralizing it with caustic soda, then drying it and making it into a powder that is used in the same way as MSG.

Now, what happens to these excitotoxins? They get in the bloodstream. They're not supposed to go through the blood/brain barrier, but they do. Aspartame and MSG get inside the brain, and both of them go to the hypothalamus. The hypothalamus is a small area in the brain that controls our appetites. The problem is that these chemicals destroy or knock out the control center. It is possible to detoxify and restore this area, but you must prevent taking these chemicals into your body and use detoxification products.

So, your appetite control center goes out of whack when you ingest these chemicals, and here you are eating more than you should and you don't even realize it. That's one of the reasons people get overweight and they don't know why they're fat. Later, we're going to talk about detoxifying, avoiding these chemicals and getting them out of your body when you can't completely avoid them. Excitotoxins are considered to be the leading cause of Alzheimer's, Parkinson's and ALS!

# Fats

"I try to avoid fats. My doctor says that we shouldn't eat fats." I hear that a lot.

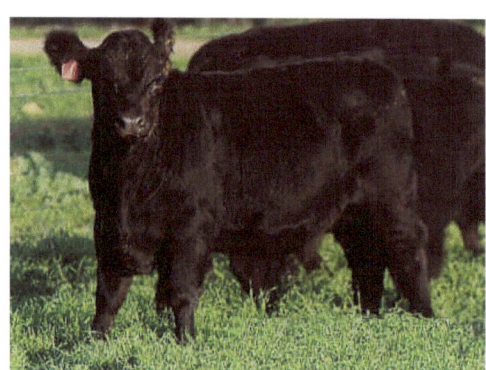

The truth is, you have to eat fats. If you don't eat some fats, your brain will do funny things like degrade into dementia. Your brain is mostly cholesterol and fats. If you don't consume some fats, you will have mental problems.

The solution is eating the right fats. We've been told for years and years that red meat was unhealthy. In fact, red meat is *not* unhealthy. Red meat is very healthy for you if it's been raised properly. You have to go back though—the feedlot beef is not healthy. Grass fed, non-chemical beef is very healthy for you. The fats in it are very safe to eat. They create or give you Omega 3 fatty acids and other essential beneficial fatty acids such as CLAs, which we need.

In fact, one of the biggest problems we have in this country is that we used to have a 1 to 1 ratio of Omega 3 to Omega 6 (Omega 6 comes from grains and vegetable oils). Now, we're running somewhere between 1 to 25 and 1 to 50, meaning more Omega 6 than Omega 3. That is very unhealthy, causing heart problems and diseases. So, we need the Omega 3. We need less Omega 6. Beef is very healthy for you, but you have to eat the right kind. There is a link on my website (www.drbobthehealthbuilder.com) where you can purchase healthy meat. The latest ploy by meat producers is injecting meat with a solution of water, salt, high fructose corn syrup, ammonium (for tenderness) and salt, removing oxygen and replacing it with carbon monoxide, and using radiation to destroy E-coli bacteria, which destroys all nutrition.

# Vegetable oils

Another thing that is not healthy for us is vegetable oil. I can't stress that enough. Vegetable oils are unhealthy. Those are the ones that are loaded with Omega 6. Vegetable oil is in everything—cookies, crackers,

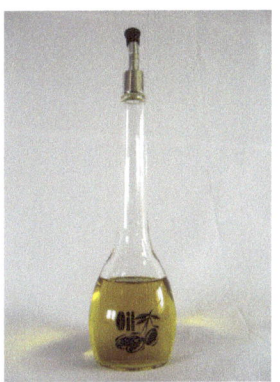

breads. Whatever you can think of, it's in there someplace. It converts to trans-fatty acids. These oils actually are really nasty when they're used as cooking oil. We'll get to those shortly, but the truth is vegetable oils are terrible.

Margarine and shortening are terrible, too. You can't believe the chemical process and solvents that go into making these very unhealthy products. Don't eat margarine (one molecule away from plastic), and don't eat vegetable oils or use shortening.

There are three oils that are considered safe. Olive oil is great to use, but cooking in it is not as good as coconut and macadamia oils. Coconut oil is very good for cooking. And then, of course, there's macadamia oil— these oils do not break down in high heat. Those three are very healthy and we should use them. Another one that is touted heavily is canola oil, but it is almost as bad as soybean or cottonseed oils. And it is genetically engineered.

# What about the American Heart Association Diet and others?

One of the things we all hear about once in awhile is the American Heart Association Diet. Honestly, if you follow that diet, you are bound to get heart disease and high blood pressure. If you think about it, since this diet came out, heart disease and blood pressure have skyrocketed. There couldn't be anything unhealthier than the American Heart Association Diet. The second one is the American Diabetic Association diet. It is horrible. If you follow that diet, you're going to get Type 2 diabetes. You have to educate yourself and you've got to stay away from these groups that are promoting their longevity, their money-making, their power, or whatever it happens to be.

I don't know if you're old enough to remember when polio was a common disease and the polio organization was raising money. When polio was beaten and the need for raising money disappeared, the organization had no place to go—no purpose. Talk about a bunch of whipped pups. All of these other organizations—the American Cancer Society, the Susan G. Komen Walk for the Cure, the American Heart Association, the American Diabetes Association—are not about to let their existence disappear. They don't want their diseases to disappear; they just don't want us to die too early.

Consequently, corporations and associations don't want cancer to go away. They don't want heart disease to go away, because then they lose their purpose, their power and their money. You really have to question these people. I've got to the point, maybe because I'm older, that I'm very cynical. Now when something comes up, the first question I ask is, "Where's the money?" When you trace these organizations, you'll find they're absolutely on the verge of being crooks.

## Companies and the government are concerned about obesity, right?

Now, do you believe that large corporations and the government are interested in you or any of your friends losing weight or healthier? If you watch television, you would think they'd be concerned, but the real truth is they couldn't care less.

There are several things to consider. We've all heard that Social Security is in trouble because we're living longer. It is true that the life expectancy now is about 77 years. But the worst thing that could happen is more people living longer and drawing on Social Security. The younger generation does not have large enough numbers, and they're not going to be able to afford to pay us when we get to retirement age. I'm talking basically about the Baby Boomers.

The government actually would like to see people start dying earlier, and obesity just may be the trick to do that. A lot of people are beginning to speculate that obesity is going to change life expectancy from 77 years average down to 72. If you change the retirement age from 65 to 68, 70 or 72, and the life expectancy goes down, guess what folks—Social Security has been saved.

Don't expect the government to care about your obesity or good health. They'll give it lip service, but in reality they don't give a flip. In fact, they're the ones that created, with the industry's input, the Food Pyramid. The Food Pyramid encourages eating carbohydrates that have no nutrition. The government is very much behind these unhealthy things. You cannot trust the powers that run everything. You have to trust yourself and the people who are speaking common sense. Remember, politicians think we are too stupid to function and they have to take care of us from womb to tomb.

And then there are, of course, companies. Do you think they want obesity to go away? Heavens no!  Drug companies love it because the fatter you get and the more diseases you have, the more drugs you have to use. You never get well because the drugs and the research are done so that you drag it out. They want you to live a long time, but they want you to do it at your expense, having to buy *their* drugs. You might be 70 years old and can't afford to eat, but they want your $1,000 to $1500 a month.  The fact is, drug companies want you to be fat.

If they could come up with some drug that may help

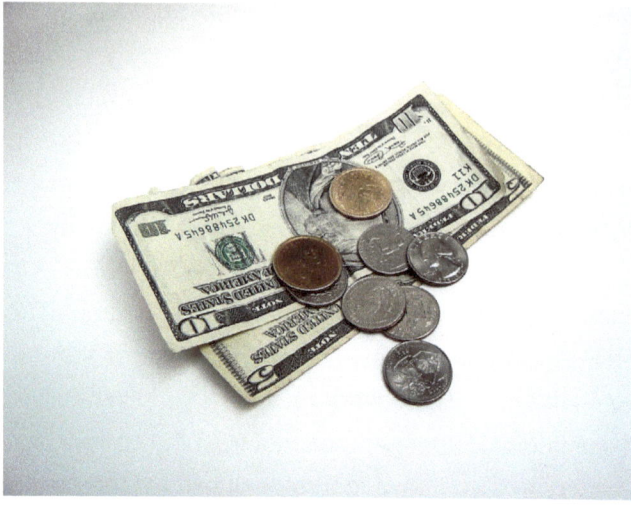

people lose weight, obviously they're going to promote it because weight loss is a large profit motive center. But these gimmicks and drugs aren't going to work. They are not going to get rid of the chemicals and provide the good food that you need, and they won't help you learn to eat healthy and lose weight. Take charge of your food and health.

Another thing about large companies—think about this: We're talking about the multi-national food companies— the ones that create the grain products, the ones that have the beef products with all the chemicals, the ones that lock chickens up and feed them a diet in which 55% is chemicals, or the pigs that are put into confinement and the mama pigs aren't allowed to turn around. All they can do is stand up, lie down, have babies, put food in one end and out the other. Talk about cruelty; this is absolutely horrible.

But these companies are not interested in you losing weight. Think about it. Fat people, no matter whether it's a little bit or a lot, eat more food. They love this. They want you to become fat. That's why there are so many chemicals in their foods. You don't expect a large company to be working in your best interest as far as helping you lose weight. They put chemicals in the food to help you gain weight. They put chemicals in to try to get you addicted to their products. On top of it, they put chemicals in food to keep you from losing weight, one of which is MSG. The other is Aspartame, because as I mentioned earlier, it goes to the hypothalamus and destroys the appetite centers so you gain weight. Don't look for these companies to give you something that's healthy.

I can remember a few years ago when all fats were declared bad. All of a sudden we had fat-free cookies. My gracious, it was nothing but carbs with no nutrition and people blew up; they got fatter with these carbs. So, don't expect these companies to solve your problems. We have to solve our own. We have to get mad as heck. I'm mad as heck and I want to solve this. I want to help other people solve it.

# Chemicals in farming

When we talk about healthy ingredients in food, food companies couldn't care less. The farming community, because of the advice from the land grant colleges, has been encouraged to use chemicals. The chemicals in farming came about after World War II. We had companies that manufactured nitrogen in the form of bombs, meaning nitrates. They didn't want to go out of business. Good gracious, they were making a ton of money during the war, so they then came up with chemical fertilizers. Then, along came the chemical warfare in World War II. That was done with organophosphates. Organophosphates were the predecessors to herbicides, pesticides and fungicides.

These companies didn't want to go out of business either; the money was great. So, that was the other part of the birth of chemical agriculture. It has nothing to do with nutrients. It has nothing to do with wholesome food. It has to do with large corporations making money. All you have to do is look at the cancer in this country. If you get into it and study it a little bit, you'll find that those chemicals used on crops are causing cancer.

It's no secret why women have breast cancer. It's no secret why men have prostrate cancer. It has to do with cosmetics/personal care products, pesticides, other chemicals and poor nutrition. Pesticides are put on all plants. The good Lord made bugs to eat crops that weren't healthy. So, we plant crops, we use chemical fertilizers that have no nutrients and the plants are ill. The Maker sends in bugs to eat what's not healthy for us, but we, in our infinite wisdom, go out and put chemicals on the plants to kill the bugs so we can eat the poor quality food.

You have to worry about what's in your food. Now, when I say worry, I don't want anybody to fret. What I'm advocating is not that difficult, it's not that expensive. It just happens to be that you've got to think ahead and plan and you can prevent a lot of the health problems, or being overweight. That's why I said earlier that with my Health Builder Program you don't have to do *everything* today. You listen to the CD or read this book multiple times and you add something new. Maybe you add a new supplement or new foods once a month to make your diet better, or to improve the food quality and make it taste better.

## Why do you need to detoxify?

One of the things we have to do is detoxify. We know there are about 1,000 chemicals in most city water supplies every day. We're talking herbicides, pesticides, fertilizers, nitrates, nitrites, hormones, antibiotics, micronized toilet paper and many more chemicals. We're referring to solvents, benzene, toluene and many other toxins. There are all sorts of chemicals and we eat them and drink them daily. The chemicals are also in the air. One of my pet peeves is that in the Dallas area they blame cars for air pollution. The truth of it is cars account for 25% of the pollution. Most of that 25% comes from older vehicles. Well, if you take the older vehicles off the road, then you have people on welfare. But, if you just leave that alone, the older vehicles die, they have to be replaced, and as they filter down from the top, the air pollution and air quality keeps getting better and better.

The problem in most communities is that it's the industry that's causing the pollution. In fact, in the Dallas area, the biggest one is Dallas-Fort Worth Airport. There is a community down south of Dallas that has concrete plants, and the government allows them to burn oils that have toxins in them. "No worry," they say. "We don't care; it's okay. It burns." But, the truth is, in that community they have one of the highest rates of Down's syndrome in a very small area. So, again, pollution is all around us, but we do have to get the toxins out of our systems. That's the key.

There are multiple ways to detoxify. But you have to find the things to get the job done without being expensive. The first thing you want to do is try to minimize toxins as much as you can. One way to do that is to use water filters. Most of the ones you see advertised on TV are just absolutely useless. Don't bother to waste your time with them. You have to get something better. You need reverse osmosis and charcoal, ultraviolet light and electrolysis to create alkaline water. There is a reference on my website (www.hightechhealth.com) for a water filtration system that is very good. Clean water will go a long ways toward detoxifying your body.

Actually, we need to have an alkaline body. A body that is slightly above 7.0 PH is less likely to get disease, particularly heart disease and cancer. So, we do need to find sources of alkaline water, and one of the best ways to get it is to filter water properly and avoid soft drinks, as they are highly acidic.

The point is to eliminate as many chemicals as possible. Once we have them in our bodies, those chemicals are one of the reasons that we're all overweight. The chemicals attach to fat cells. You can starve yourself. You can get way down on weight and then you blow the diet and it all bounces back. The reason is the fat cells are still there and they're attached to the toxic chemicals. But if you can get rid of the toxic chemicals, then you can shrink fat cells forever so that it's actually harder to gain weight back later.

Besides detoxifying with prevention, we also have to detoxify with products. One of the products that I'm very fond of is from a personal friend over in Fort Worth,

Texas, who has developed a product called humates. I started using it on my farm to detoxify the soil and it worked well. Then I found out about the version for animals, and then about the version for humans. When I started losing weight, part of my program had to be detoxification. I use humates, which is available for purchase on my website (www.drbobthehealthbuilder.com). It's not overly expensive by any means. One capsule a day will take care of detoxification, but it really helps to be healthy. At the same time, it adds trace minerals.

Trace minerals are better when you get them through plants, but chelated is okay. I advocate the humate because it has multiple trace minerals, particularly calcium, and they're chelated so your body can absorb them properly. I also like to get trace minerals through plant sources, and we'll get to that soon.

One of the ways to detoxify is through using a sauna. The idea of this goes back to the 1950s. I'm not advocating the church that he started, but anybody who knows of L. Ron Hubbard knows that he started a church. Hubbard's church attracted a number of people who were down and out. I'm talking about drug addicts, alcoholics and what have you. I have no idea what prompted Mr. Hubbard to detoxify, but his theory was that if you have toxic chemicals in your body from these drugs and you try to quit, those toxic chemicals are still in there and are a kind of irritant. It will always make you want to go back because they are in your system, so Hubbard advocated hot saunas.

At that time there were only steam saunas. But people who got involved with him went to saunas and detoxified to get these chemicals out of their systems. Many of them were so appreciative that they got involved with the church. Incidentally, the church was the Church of Scientology. Again, I'm not advocating that; I'm just telling you what happened.

Today, we have better saunas. The main saunas for detoxification are Far Infrared Saunas. You can control the temperature. You can control the time. The saunas with the far infrared penetrate through the skin and help release toxic chemicals. I have talked to smokers who went into these saunas. The first two or three times they came out they had brown stuff all over their skin. That was the nicotine that was coming out of their systems. Go to www.hightechhealth.com where you can find out all kinds of information. One is about water; they have a really good filter. The other one is about the Far Infrared Saunas.

I have mentioned the word *excitotoxins* before when I talked about Equal and MSG. I mentioned that excitotoxins can get in the bloodstream and into the brain; they go past the blood/brain barrier and go in to the hypothalamus. These toxins cause more problems than just weight gain. Aspartame is probably the leading cause of migraine headaches in this country today. It has been known to cause brain tumors and brain defects in children.

There is a really good book about Aspartame written by H.R. Roberts, who is an MD. He wrote the book in the late 80's. This knowledge has been out there for 15, 16 or 17 years, and more and more information has been compiled. In fact, when Roberts wrote his book, a lot of the information he got were reports that had been sent by the average person into the FDA. The FDA has completely ignored those pleas, or cries, for help with problems caused by Aspartame.

## Trace minerals

Trace minerals are essential for your body. We need vitamins, we need minerals, we need amino acids and enzymes to make various chemical functions work in our bodies. That's the one time I use the word "chemical" and it's not bad. Our bodies are massive chemical factories. If you take in the right ingredients, you get the right products back out. But you have to have the right stuff, and the right stuff includes trace minerals. If we don't have trace minerals, then our factories will go awry. You may end up with diabetes, arthritis, heart disease, cancer, multiple sclerosis, autoimmune disease and many more serious health problems. A 2006 book by Charles Walters, *Minerals for the Genetic Code* (www.acresusa.com), traces every disease to the lack of trace minerals.

That's why one of the statements I put on my website is that, in this country, 6.5 people out of every 10 have a degenerative disease. You may remember Linus Pauling, PhD; he was probably the only man who won two Nobel Prizes in two different areas of science. This man was really sharp in the causes of disease. He said that almost every disease can be traced to the absence of trace minerals.

You need trace minerals and you need them in a form that your body can absorb – either chelated or preferably phyto—plant derived. Remember calcium citrate? That's the metallic form and therefore not absorbable, so you can continue to have osteoporosis because the calcium is not going into your body in the proper way. The best trace minerals are *Dr Bob's Total Ocean Nutrition* (TON) minerals. These are phyto-minerals—from kelp, plankton and other plants in the ocean off the coast of Australia —and ionic, therefore they are readily absorbable by our bodies. Our bodies pick up toxic chemicals when the right minerals are not available and this causes disease The thyroid is a perfect example. Without iodine, which is not present in our food supply, the body takes fluoride and bromine into the thyroid gland to cause disease. The good news is that if you take Dr. Bob's TON, the iodine in our product will expel the fluoride and bromine from the thyroid and return it to good health.

Remember: "You don't have to wealthy to be healthy," which is why *Dr Bob's TON* minerals are not only great for your health, but inexpensive, too, at $24.97 for a two-month supply per person.

## Fish oils

We need Omega 3s. I've mentioned it before. Where can you get it? The easiest way to supplement is to use fish oils. The problem is that almost all the fish oils, both in the grocery stores as well as even health food stores, come from far away places. It's processed, put into containers, shipped, stored in warehouses and finally manufactured. The oils oxidize and there is no nutrition left. It's not a good product, and to get a therapeutic dose you would have to take 20 capsules per day. When you consider the price, you realize it's not a good bargain (100 caps is a 5 day supply). On top of this, I have just discovered that companies are mixing fish oil with vegetable oils to dilute the product. With this you get poor oil and trans fatty acids.

You need to ask where the source is. Who makes it? What's the quality? I offer a product on my website that I call Dr Bob's Total Ocean Nutrition (TON)—Salmon Oil. It is loaded with virgin salmon oil, which is full of Omega 3s—and not only that—the EPA, the DHA and other beneficial fatty acids are also present. You want to look for sources that you can trust, and there aren't many trustworthy products available. Our oil is caught in cold environment, taken to port in the cold, minimal cold processing, packaged in cold, sealed, and then sent to the US.

There is a product on the market that contains shark liver oil, and it also has the Omega 3s from other fish sources. The problem is it's very expensive because it's sold through multi-level marketing. The products that I have are less expensive, and you can buy them from my website. You'll find that the shark liver oil will be very expensive; however, a bottle of *Dr Bob's TON—Salmon Oil* is just $19.97 per bottle for 45 days for most people (I also occasionally run specials on the website.)

There are a number of diseases that are affected by the lack of Omega 3s, DHA, and EPA, such as ADD, ADHD, depression, arthritis and heart disease. With depression, one of the primary causes, besides toxic chemicals, is the lack of beneficial fatty acids. These products are important in a lot of different ways. Also, heart disease can be vastly improved with quality beneficial fatty acids.

# Is chicken good for me?

Doctors advise patients (on TV and in offices), "Don't eat red meat, it's not healthy. Eat chicken." Well, okay, let's go back for a second. Beef in feedlots is loaded with five hormones, steroids, antibiotics and other chemicals left over from worming products, plus arsenic from the chicken manure that they feed the cows. The cattle stand around and contaminate each other. They ingest herbicides and pesticides from the grain they're fed. So you're told that chicken is better.

But stop and think about chicken. Chickens are put into a building. There are thousands of them together. Their beaks are taken off, so they will not kill each other. Fifty-five percent of their diet is chemicals. One of the chemicals is my favorite, and I don't mean a positive favorite, but a bad favorite: arsenic. The management companies give the chickens arsenic for five weeks before they're slaughtered. Five days before the chickens are slaughtered they remove the arsenic, and they want you to believe that the arsenic is no longer present. The truth is, even though they take it out of the food, the arsenic is still in the manure on the floor and these chicken houses are only cleaned out after every four or five batches of chickens grown. That means the chickens are walking around on the arsenic. So arsenic is in chickens today, along with hormones, antibiotics and other chemicals. My point is that beef and chicken are unhealthy when purchased in a store. Healthy beef and chicken is great, but you need to find a local source that raises these proteins in a healthy manner—to your good health!

Now, of course, there is also goat meat and lamb. Cloven hoofed animals, or those with multiple stomachs, should not eat grains because the grain is unhealthy, and it destroys the Omega 3s and other beneficial fatty acids. Herbicides and pesticides in the feed grains are also toxic.

# Aren't eggs high in cholesterol?

I really like eggs. Eggs are very good for you. We've been told that if you eat eggs that the cholesterol from the eggs causes cholesterol in your body. There couldn't be anything further from the truth. There has never, ever, been one study to prove this statement. Now, on the other hand, what do you get when you buy eggs in the grocery store? First of all, when you buy them and they're listed as fresh, they're at least 30 days old and most likely 90 to 180 days old. That means they've been sitting around someplace, maybe in a cooler, maybe in heat, maybe in a truck. But, they're hardly fresh.

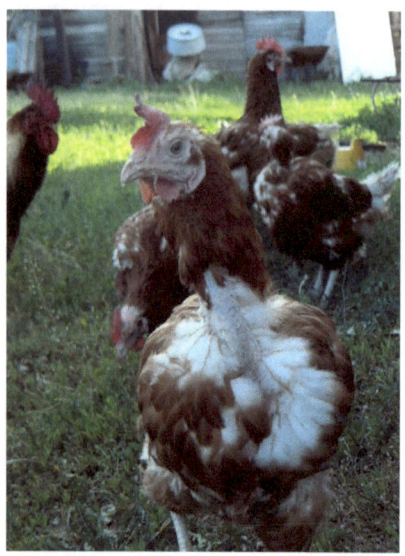

The chickens that lay the eggs are put into boxes. The chickens are hardly allowed to move and the farmers give them a chemical diet. I had a patient in the office years ago and he said, "Well, I prefer my eggs, because I know what they eat." I said, "No, I prefer chickens out on a pasture eating grass and bugs." He said, "Well, bugs aren't healthy for them." Well, the truth is, they are. The good Lord put chickens on earth to help get rid of the bugs. They do it well, and they convert into very healthy products.

Eggs are healthy for you. The bottom line is you need to buy them someplace else. Buy them from a local farmer. We have people all over the United States who are beginning to raise healthy foods. Look for these people; seek them out, or just find somebody who has a chicken yard. There are people who still raise chickens and sell country eggs. There are sources of fresh wholesome foods and it's not that difficult to find them.

Remember, cholesterol is created in your liver from eating grains, sugar, High Fructose Corn Syrup and other carbohydrates—not from eating cholesterol.

# My doctor tells me to eat lots of fish

Fish, unfortunately, is one of the worst things you can eat. If you can buy wild salmon from Alaska or from Norway, or some place that we know is safe, that's great. But the truth is, most of the fish today is farm raised. The people farming fish know that the food they give them is loaded with mercury, PCBs and Dioxins, but they do it anyway. They grind up small fish into a meal and feed the fish that are raised in confinement areas. These little fish are also loaded with herbicides and pesticides found in the water they are raised in. Folks, this is not a good thing. If you want to eat salmon, it is good, but make sure it came from Alaska or another safe area of the world—not from a farm.

Incidentally, there have been some restaurants and grocery stores that have been singled out as lying to their customers, saying that they were serving wild salmon when in fact they were not. It was farm raised.

# Working out

A lot of people advocate that you need to go to the gym to lose weight. Don't get me wrong, I'm not opposed to exercise if it's done in moderation (it is essential). But to go to the gym and work your brains out until your body falls apart is stupid. Lifting weights to tone up is wonderful. Walking on a treadmill or stair stepper is wonderful, but don't exercise to lose weight. Eat right, avoid chemical foods and exercise to improve your health, not to wear out your joints and other body parts.

Walking around your block is excellent. Walking is wonderful exercise. Personally, I prefer riding a bike. I don't do it often enough, but I do it when I can. What I like about the bike is, 1) I pedal a lot, which is good for my knees and ankles, but 2) if I go up a hill, I walk because I want to get the exercise for my ankles and my feet. For me, I love to go 8 to 10 miles. I have different trails and favorite places that I go to. I have farm animals that come up the fence and get their heads scratched. I have a couple of donkeys that come up, and I stop and rub them between the ears and take a little break. Or if it's really hot, I stop under a tree, catch my breath, drink a little water and then go on.

So, you want to exercise, but you want to do it in moderation. Don't try to lose weight by trying to exercise it off. You want to get rid of the chemicals, you want to eat right, and you want to exercise because it's important. But don't wear your body out.

# What about "brown bagging" it?

What do you do as far as lunch? Do you brown bag it? It's not a bad idea. I don't like to do it, but you can do it. Another thing for lunch is take a banana and an apple. Bananas that are organic are harder to find, but you can find them. The good news about a banana is that when you strip the skin off, it doesn't have as many toxic chemicals as an apple that was sprayed with pesticides. You should buy organic apples. If you don't have any choice, then buy apples, but clean them with some kind of mild soapy solution and rinse them thoroughly so you get rid of those toxic chemicals that are on there, despite the fact that farmers may tell you they're not sprayed.

In fact, there was a law passed a few years ago that forbids anybody to publicly report that fruit has had a pesticide sprayed to prevent bug damage. Maybe you remember the alarm caused when use of a pesticide made the news 8 to 10 years ago—the sale of apples dropped, and growers in the northwest US almost went broke. Instead of growing healthy apples, they got the law changed.

Take fresh fruits and vegetables when you brown bag. One thing I didn't mention earlier when I was talking about buying organic fresh fruits and vegetables—and you really need to get them organic—is that fruit trees have longer roots, and they go deeper in the soil. So, you're more likely to get trace minerals out of fruits than you are out of vegetables. That's why you want vegetables that are grown with trace minerals, because they don't have the ability to go down deep, deep in the soil and bring the trace minerals up where they can be used by the plants. Remember, our good health depends on minerals, macro and trace.

I admit that I don't like to brown bag it. I do carry fruit, and sometimes I eat it in the office in the middle of the afternoon. Sometimes I'm starved to death when I leave the office. I've saved an apple and I'll eat it on the way home. However, mostly what we do at the office is buy salads. It's not that difficult. I don't want croutons, or strips of tortilla chips in it, and I try to eat a very minimum in terms of dressings. I prefer the Paul Newman dressings because they do not use genetically engineered canola oil or soybean oil. His products are a cut above the others, who make dressings that are mostly chemicals. Ranch dressing may be the worst; read the labels.

Unfortunately, Paul Newman has started putting products in plastic containers. One of the important things that people need to know is plastic, wraps, bottles, and containers, infuses gases into the food or drinks that you consume causing depression, cancer and estrogen imitation. Meat and fruits in grocery stores that are wrapped in plastic film and styrene bottoms are horrible for out gassing. You should never drink something hot in a Styrofoam cup. It's just like drinking styrene. Chemicals from plastics will cause depression and cancer, and also they imitate hormones. Not a good thing for anyone and particularly for young girls and boys.

# If I have to eat out, how do I avoid some of these toxins and grains?

When you are traveling you have to eat somewhere. One of the things I do is buy a hamburger. It's not great. I know the meat has chemicals in it, but I try to minimize the bad things. I may get a hamburger, but I will get it without mayonnaise. Mayonnaise is loaded with soybean oils and that means herbicides and pesticides. I don't use ketchup because of the sugars and stuff that are in it. I do use mustard. I eat the vegetables, meaning the lettuce, onions and tomatoes. I throw the bread away. I didn't say it was perfect, but it's a way to get by when traveling. If I eat breakfast on the road I will get an omelet without toast and pancakes. For dinner I will get a steak (without seasonings to avoid MSG) with a sweet potato or steamed veggies without bread.

What happens if you're out and somebody wants chicken? Well, again, I understand there's a problem. There are all kinds of chemicals in chicken. What you need to know, though, is that most of the chemicals in chicken are in the skin. If I go someplace and there is chicken, I know I don't want the vegetable oil. But where does the vegetable oil go? It's absorbed into the skin and it's absorbed into the breading that's on the chicken. So, I throw away all the breading, all the skin; I take the meat out, which has been cooked around with the vegetable oils, but they aren't in the meat. Again, it's not perfect, but we're not in a perfect world.

There are a number of other things you can do when you're out, but those are just some of the basics. Sometimes you're in a group and somebody wants pizza. The good Lord knows pizza is not full of benefits. First of all, the dough is horrible. It is stripped of all nutrition. There is a lot of MSG used on pizzas. But, again, if you're in a group and you don't want to look too silly, what I do is get a pizza, and I will have extra cheese and meat put on it—not the sauce because there's MSG in that. Then, I'll just eat the topping. You can take half a pizza, eat the topping and you're not overloaded at all, and you feel full.

Another thing I love is Tex-Mex food. I go to Mexican restaurants at times, but I don't eat chips because remember, the chips are made out of corn. It is probably genetically engineered. Also, they've been fried in oils. So, here's what I do, which kind of looks silly, but I love salsa, and for the most part salsa doesn't have much that's bad in it. There are usually tomatoes, onions, peppers, cilantro and things like that, so I eat the salsa with the chip, but I use the chip over and over again. If the chip starts to get a little soggy, I just throw it away.

I also love fajita nachos. I know they're not the best. I know they use MSG in the meat, but I don't eat the chips, so if I order them, I get them with cheese and

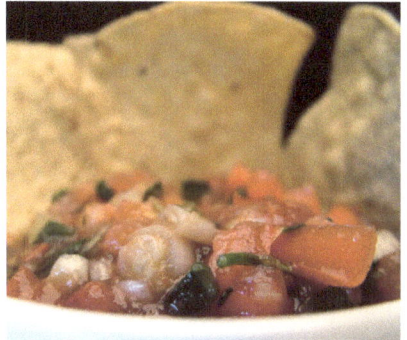

frijoles, which are refried beans. I scrape the topping off and don't eat the chips. Again, it's not perfect, but sometimes you're out and you can't avoid it. You have to do something and you have to try to eat as best as you possibly can. Remember, I'm still taking the humates to detoxify and I am eating well at home. Unfortunately chicken, beef and pork is being pumped up with a solution of water, MSG, salt, HFCS and sometimes ammonia.

# What if I blow my healthy eating?

A lot of people will "fall off the healthy food wagon." They feel guilty for getting off their diets, lose their interest and gain their weight back. There is a way around that with my Health Builder Program. I blow it once in a while when my wife and I go out to dinner. Now, I try to order a steak cooked without their seasonings because the seasonings are loaded with MSG.

I will buy vegetables instead of a potato; I never eat white potatoes. A potato is a very unhealthy product for the amount of carbs they produce. It's very fattening, just nothing but carbs. A lot of restaurants today have sweet potatoes, so I'll order a sweet potato with real butter, never margarine. One of the restaurants we go to has French fried onion rings. I know it's terrible, and I shouldn't do it, but indulging once every three or four months is not going to destroy my health.

When you eat healthy, eating junk once in a while does not destroy your weight loss program, and you don't need to feel guilty.

# Butter is bad for me, right?

You are commonly told, and I mentioned this earlier, that butter is unhealthy for you. Butter is actually very *healthy* for you, if it is organic from non-pasteurized milk. There are two choices: Horizon and Organic Valley. Or find a local dairy that produces healthy butter. You may have to look in a few stores to find organic milk, butter and cottage cheese, but it will be worth your efforts. There is a problem with organic milk because the cows are fed grains. It would be better if they were grass fed, but it is almost impossible to find grass-fed dairy products. If you can't find grass-fed products, you can get organic, which is much better than store–bought, regular milk (or the "white liquid substance") or butter.

Butter (saturated fats are very healthy if they come from healthy sources and consumed in moderation) is wonderful for you, tastes great and it is healthy. Remember, you should never eat margarine or butter substitutes.

# The five worst foods

One of my favorite subjects is "The Five Worst Foods You Can Eat." There is a doctor in Illinois who advocates this, and he's absolutely right. The five worst things you can eat are:

➡ French fries

- Chips
- Doughnuts
- Soft drinks
- Seafood

Because you've read this book, you understand what I'm talking about with the fish. It's because of the mercury, the dioxins and the PCBs.

Without a doubt, if you pick up a bag of chips and look at what's in it, and you can't pronounce or spell most of it, you shouldn't eat it.

French fries—terrible! White potatoes have almost no nutrition. Vegetable oils are terrible trans fatty acids. Doughnuts are nothing but sugar and vegetable oil! Soft drinks are horrible. No one should ever drink a soft drink. It's bad enough that you drink ones with sugar, which don't exist in the United States except in a very limited quantity. Back in the early 80s, soft drink companies were using sugar in soft drinks. But because the government had tariffs to keep the price of imported sugar high, corporations started using corn syrup, which is cheap. Therefore, corporations substitute sugar with corn syrup. Sugar will trigger your insulin system, and you'll get to the point where you have had enough.  But with the corn syrup, that won't happen. People end up drinking more soft drinks with corn syrup.

Also, don't forget the phosphoric acid, which eats away the lining of your stomach. There isn't anything good about soft drinks. Of course, as I mentioned before, the diet soft drinks are even worse because most of them are made with Equal, although we're now getting some made with Splenda. Those just are not products you should be drinking.

I want to add two more foods to that list of five. I know kids ask for it, and it's difficult to avoid their pleadings, but macaroni and cheese is terrible. First of all, the macaroni is extruded. That means no nutrition, zip, and zero. On top of it, they have cheese. Well, read the label and you'll find out it's not cheese. It's a cheese substitute, it's a cheese food. Most of it is just toxic chemicals—some of those 3,000 they put in various foods today. This cheese never saw a cow!

If you just have to give your child macaroni and cheese, at least go to the health food store and buy non-extruded macaroni. It is not loaded with herbicides, pesticides and other chemicals. Then, use real cheese—I mean real cheese! That's hard to find in grocery stores today, but you can find it (generally, imported cheese comes from countries that don't use bovine growth hormones). That's a much better alternative than buying what's in those boxes.

The seventh one is pizza. The breads, the flour, or whatever you want to call it, in the pizza is terrible. Pizza is very, very fattening because it's all carbs and no nutrition and packed with various chemicals in the dough and in the sauce.

Maybe you can make a whole-wheat pizza. You should be able to make a healthy sauce. At least, try to do the right thing. Don't give your kids what comes from the stores. Don't eat what comes from the purveyors of pizza.

## What do you do for snacks?

Everybody has to snack on something. I come home from work and I'm starved. One of my snacks is cheese. Again, we've been told that it's very unhealthy. The bottom line is that's just not true. Cheese is wonderful if you buy good cheese—and there's the problem. Most of the name brand cheeses in the stores are terrible. I have found that there are some stores I can go to that carry cheeses from outside the United States, and it's considerably better because Europe doesn't use all the chemicals that we do.

I also have a source that I've put in this book. Pretty much everybody's heard about the Amish. The Amish live a very simple life, a very Christian life and a very secluded life. They don't use all the chemicals the corporations do. I have a source in Ohio where I can buy cheeses made by Amish families, and it is wonderful cheese. They particularly make some of the best Swiss cheese that I've ever, ever eaten. Fortunately, there are sources where you can get healthy cheese, but, again, we're talking about cows that didn't have all the chemicals pumped into them, and they didn't have all the fertilizers in the grasses they ate.

Another healthy food is walnuts. They are good because they have Omega 3s. Frankly, I'm just not a connoisseur of walnuts. I will eat some occasionally, but it's just not one of my favorites. I do love pecans, and I have found sources where I can buy them that do not have a lot of chemicals. Besides, if you put a lot of the chemicals in a pecan orchard, you're going to kill the trees. So, for the most part, you're going to have a lot less chemicals in nuts then you will other things.

I happen to love pecans that are roasted. A lot of people roast them with salt. If you use a good salt, which we'll discuss, that's okay. Personally, I just like to have them roasted and they're wonderful. I also like to snack on cauliflower, mini carrots, celery and broccoli—without dressings.

# Genetically modified organisms

Another thing we have to discuss is GMO. That stands for Genetically Modified Organisms. There are different terms, but GMO is one of the most common ones. Genetically Engineered is another term. Genetically engineered foods are sometimes referred to as Franken foods. You remember who Frankenstein was? He was put together of various parts and then brought to life. Well, the reason we call them Franken foods is you take the good crops and shoot genes into these things, and you create body parts.

Well, it's not exactly body parts—but you create other problems. There are a lot of these out there. I mentioned earlier that soybeans are 95% genetically engineered. The main reason they are genetically engineered is so they would tolerate more herbicides and pesticides, but particularly the herbicides. That means you have more cancer-causing ingredients than in non-organic, non-GEO soybeans.

You cannot escape soybeans. You just start reading labels and you'll find them in everything you buy. It's a perversion, but the FDA says that it's a health food and that it prevents cancer. The FDA is letting soy food manufacturers claim health benefits that are just not true. This isn't miso and it isn't tofu, and it's not from

Japan, where they have some semblance of not wanting to use chemicals, and particularly genetically engineered ones. Find out the source of what you're eating, but don't eat soybeans.

Franken foods—the companies don't like that name—create all sorts of problems. Remember, Franken foods are genetically engineered foods. They were not manufactured for health. They were manufactured by companies trying to destroy the good foods so we have to buy their trash foods and so that they can control the world's population.

They are exporting toxic garbage to other countries as well. The latest one is South Africa. If you go to my website at www.drbobthehealthbuilder.com, I did an article that was an interview with Jeffrey Smith. He wrote a book called *Seeds of Deception*. I published the interview that was done in South Africa. We're going to see that South Africa is a big experiment for all of these toxic foods, and they're going to use more of them. We're going to see what happens to their population in the next two to three generations.

# Herbicides and pesticides

Herbicides and pesticides are pervasive in our food system, and they need to be removed or avoided as much as possible. A female's normal hormones and estrogens are about 500 parts per trillion. Men's are about 50 parts per trillion. When plants are already unhealthy due to pesticides, the bugs should eat them up. But instead, the farmers spray them with pesticides. Sometimes, it's only an ounce or two per acre. But, the fact is the pesticides imitate estrogens at 31,000 parts per trillion.

It doesn't take a brain surgeon to figure out that if you put 31,000 parts per trillion on corn, on wheat, on soy beans and then you eat it, even though you're not going to get the whole 31,000 parts per trillion, a woman will be getting a whole lot more than 500 parts per trillion. For a man, you're getting a whole lot more than 50 parts per trillion.

Breast cancer—I've said it before—is caused by pesticides and other toxic chemicals. Prostrate cancer is caused by pesticides and other toxic chemicals. We've got to learn to avoid the products that contain toxic chemicals.

## Fertilizers

I did an interview with a woman by the name of Patti Martin up in Quincy, Washington, on my radio show several years ago. One of the things they discovered in

Quincy (and this has been going on all over the United States and is not unique to that area) was that industrial companies have leftover products. When I say products, it may be mercury, lead, cadmium, arsenic, antimony, aluminum and other heavy metal or toxic chemicals.

If they can convince the powers that be that this leftover is a trace mineral, then they sell it to the fertilizer companies. The fertilizer company uses these chemicals as fillers. Then, unbeknownst to the farmer, he spreads it on his fields. He harvests the crops and, guess what? You get to ingest lead, or mercury, or aluminum, or whatever, in your food. When you ingest these products, they cause disease-related problems. There was even an incident of lead showing up in French fries.

One thing we talked about earlier was trace minerals. If you're not getting trace minerals, then some of these toxic chemicals will actually replace the trace minerals you ought to have, which then causes a breakdown in your body. In particular, thyroid disease is one of the more common problems in this country. There is almost no iodine in our food today, and without iodine the thyroid will take up fluoride or bromine to create illness and shut down the thyroid gland. The good news is that if you supplement to get iodine, the iodine will push the fluoride or bromine out and your thyroid will recover.

Another thing we need to know is that when you have a garden and you buy fertilizer, it's not the same as the farmer buying umpteen tons and putting it out. It's in a plastic bag. What's in that bag? Most people think its fertilizer, but the truth is over 50 % is filler. What's the filler? It is

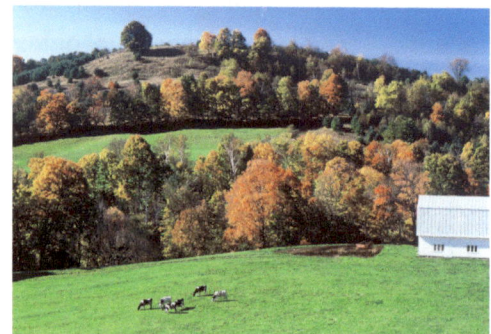

industrial waste. If it's an inert industrial waste, probably not as toxic, but that bag you're buying could be loaded with toxic chemicals, industrial waste, heavy metals or just a neutral industrial waste.

The truth is, you'll never know what's in there unless you want to pay good dollars for a chemical analysis. By then, what was the purpose of it? Besides, organic fertilizers are so much less expensive. They grow better, and better tasting, crops. You need to raise organic or Wholistic Agriculture™ crops (www.eatwild.com) or understand how to find healthy products.

# Supplements

You need the right chemical factory in your body to be healthy and lose weight. I've mentioned it before. That's the Omega 3s and other essential beneficial fatty acids, and trace minerals. Detoxification is essential, and there are several ways to do this. Trace minerals alone are the first and best way. Using *Dr Bob's Total Ocean Nutrition—Minerals* is the best starting point, and it is inexpensive.

Another product that goes a step beyond my minerals is *Dr Bob's Humates FP*. This product has trace minerals, but for detoxification it contains fulvic acid and humic acid that help chelate heavy metals and other toxins so the body can dispose of these unwanted products. You can go to www.drbobthehealthbuilder.com to get more information about these products. Humates also help to restore the immune system. With humates you can put herpes into remission, prevent hangovers from drinking alcohol and help to change a positive pap smear into a negative pap smear. Humates also help detoxify the liver.

Dr. Murray discovered years ago that mammals and fish in the ocean almost never had cancer, whereas on land, people and fresh water fish have a lot of cancer. That was because of the trace minerals that provided the nutrition. There are 92 trace minerals in seawater that I use as fertilizer. We probably don't need 92, but tell me which ones do we need and which ones we don't.

If ocean water is put on the soil, quality food products— plants—will provide healthy vitamins and minerals.

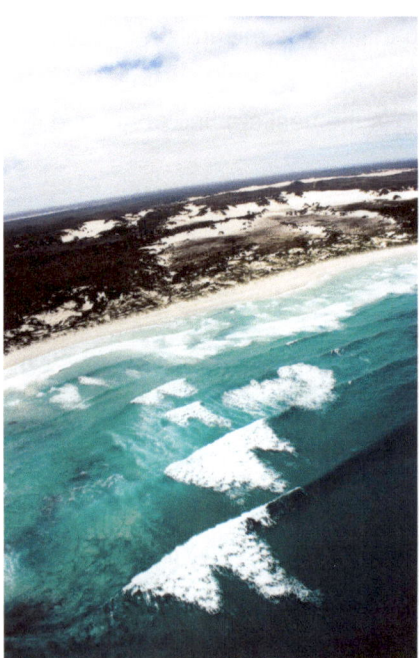

Wheat grass, grown in your house on stainless steel trays, is a wonderful source of nutrition. The seawater is very inexpensive. A gallon of seawater will last you years. You can buy red organic wheat seed from various safe sources. You put this product on the seed and wheat grass will be the result. You can actually chew the wheat grass or juice it, and you get the all the vitamins and minerals your body will ever need.

Remember, I mentioned earlier about the phyto-minerals. Phyto is plant derived and this is where the healthy wheat grass or garden vegetables can come into your food supply. There are some people who sell wheat grass capsules that are good. They don't have the 92 trace minerals, but they're organic and they're good. I recommend either buying or growing wheat grass juice or wheat grass capsules for convenience. However, growing your own vegetables is best or seeking a local producer with whom you can develop a personal relationship so you know the quality that you are getting can't be beat.

I had mentioned earlier about water and I'm going to touch on it briefly. We want it purified as much as we can. We don't want to use the cheap TV advertised filters because they don't work very effectively. Go to the HighTech Health" link on my site and check out their filter unit as it may be the best in the market place. They also have a FIR sauna that is excellent for further detoxification.

# What about salt?

I haven't touched on salt very much other than the fact that saying salt is bad. Most of the salt is bad, particularly on chips and French fries and stuff like that because all of the goodness was stripped out of it. But there are salts that are very, very beneficial, loaded with trace minerals. In this book there are resources for you to be able to find healthy products. One of them is Redmond Mineral Company, probably one of the finest in the world.

You do need salt. In fact, Redmond has testimonials of people who had high blood pressure and decided to switch over to Redmond salt with 70 trace minerals. After they started using it, their blood pressure changed to completely normal. The salt was replacing the trace minerals they weren't getting. It allowed the manufacturing process in their bodies to be able to function well. The secret treatment to cure high blood pressure is to consume magnesium and calcium in a proper balance of other minerals. Sea salt is not always good for you. Many corporations remove the trace minerals from sea salt to give us a product that is not any better than what is sold in grocery stores

# Will this "eat healthy" program work for everybody?

Yes, it will. This program will work for everybody! It will make everybody feel better, lose weight, or at least be healthier.

# Dr. Atkins

I'm often asked, "What do you think about Dr. Atkins?" Well, I don't totally agree with Dr. Atkins and his diet that advocates no carbs at all. You can tell because I've already talked about that. But one thing about Dr. Atkins that's wonderful is that he was the first doctor of any import or notoriety who said, "I can cure heart disease. I can cure high blood pressure. I can cure diabetes."

I want to tell you that put shivers down the spines of medicine and drug companies. These people are not into anyone getting cured. Now in all fairness, there are a lot of doctors out there who don't believe that. They believe they can help people and make their lives better. But, medicine in general is controlled by drug companies. The official policy is they don't want anybody to get well. They want these diseases to hang around because of all the money they can make.

To give you an idea, if you're diagnosed with Type 2 diabetes by your doctor, you represent about $250,000 to $300,000 in his pocket before you die. There's not a lot of motivation to really change courses. That's why *you* have to do it and find the doctors who are willing to help you. We have references for you, so you won't have any trouble finding doctors around the country who are looking to make you feel better, make you healthier and help you survive longer. The main thing is the quality of your life will be better.

Dr. Atkins has been chastised by the drug companies and the medical community for what he did. The truth of what he said was that grains and other carbohydrates cause Type 2 diabetes, cholesterol, heart disease, high blood pressure and a lot of other problems. By eliminating carbohydrates, many people got well and he was very successful at it. Again, I think it's a bit extreme because we really do need some carbs. That's why I advocate the right carbohydrates.

But Dr. Atkins deserves a big round of applause and credit. There were people who tried to destroy him after he died. The man slipped on ice and had a brain injury and he died from that. He was not fat and obese, other than he was possibly pumped full of drugs and chemicals before he died. This man should be taken seriously. He was not the villain the drug corporations have been trying to make him out to be.

## Vegetarian diets

Another topic is vegetarian diets. Vegetarians for the most part are the unhealthiest people you will ever encounter in your life. Most of them are doing it because they don't believe in eating animals, and that's certainly their right. But they're not eating right. They're not getting the amino acids they need. They're not getting the enzymes they need. For the most part, the ones I've known, most of them eat junk food. Most of them are overweight or they starve themselves. But they're overweight nonetheless. They eat a lot of grains like cookies, pizzas and pastas. These are some of the worst junk foods available.

There are a few cultures that I don't agree with on a religious basis, such as the Buddhists. But they do know how to supplement properly and they are healthy. But for the most part, vegetarians do not follow a healthy eating life style.

Again to remind you, my Health Builder Program is not hard to follow. But if you read this book over and over again, you'll pick up bits and pieces and put it together. Over a period of time, you'll be healthier. When I first started, I lost a lot of weight in the beginning. That was very encouraging. After that, the weight loss slowed. But one thing I knew, or noticed, was that I didn't have the urge for sugars and junk foods. In fact, for me to even think about a soft drink I get nauseated.

As I have gone on with this program, I eat less. I'm eating to live, not living to eat. I don't have strong cravings for things. I will admit once in a while a piece of chocolate is great. I don't buy the chocolate candy bars because there is so much other junk stuff in them. I don't have to pig out because I don't have the desire to do that.

# Alcohol

I didn't mention alcohol yet, and we should do that. There have certainly been studies that small amounts of alcohol are not harmful and can be beneficial. Wine is probably best. I'll drink a beer maybe once every two or three months. But you can't drink two or three beers every night. You have to give that up. Remember, when you drink alcohol it converts to sugar and will increase your body weight.

Certainly, if you want a glass of wine or shot of whiskey once in a while, I don't see that's a big deal. I'm not going to do it very often. In fact, I love Wild Turkey and cola, but the bottom line is I just don't have the desire for them because I've got to the point where thinking about colas makes me almost sick. I haven't had a drink in almost four years.

# Read the label!

Eating and drinking should be in moderation. Watch and read what your labels say. When you pick up ranch dressing, look at all the chemicals in it. When you pick up chips, look at all the chemicals in them. My wife bought a soup from a well-known national company that was broccoli and cheese. There wasn't any cheese in it! It was all cheese substitute and chemicals. There were more chemicals in it than there was broccoli. Read labels—if you can't spell it or pronounce it don't eat it.

Watch your labels and stay away from the bad stuff. If you have headaches, think about these toxic chemicals that are in all these prepared foods. Try to prepare as much food as you can for yourself. Buy organic and/or local when you can. That's important. Local food is always healthier than long distance food.

## Summary

This is the summary of my Health Builder Program, and I want it to be as simple as possible: Remember "What the Big Companies Don't Want You to Know." Believe me, the government and big corporations don't want you to know what I'm revealing to you. There are several tips that you need to discover.

- Supplement properly.

- You must detoxify.

- Stay away from MSG, Aspartame and hydrolyzed vegetable (or soy) proteins. These are excitotoxins that damage the brain in two ways. One way is to damage the appetite control center to cause obesity, and the other damages the part of the brain that creates Alzheimer's, Parkinson's disease and ALS.

- Don't eat white. That means white sugar, white potatoes, white anything. If it's white, it has no nutrition in it. The average person ate 6 pounds of sugar per year 100 years ago and today that is 175 pounds of high fructose corn syrup. This is a cause of most disease.

➡ No soy beans! Only eat fermented soy, as in tofu. All soy is unhealthy and it cause disease like cancer. When a label says soybean, soy lecithin or soy whatever, don't eat it.

➡ No corn products. Corn is not a vegetable, it's a grain. It's fattening. I recommend a no-grain or minimal-grain eating program.

➡ Look at all your labels. You've got to read the labels to avoid the chemicals.

➡ If you're out and you need to eat, minimize. Eat fruits, vegetables and salads mostly. If it's a hamburger you gotta have, throw the bread away. Stay away from the secret sauce. Stay away from the ketchup and eat the meat. It's not too bad. Chicken—strip everything off but the meat, just eat the meat.

➡ Don't use milk, particularly store bought milk. Use organic when you have to have milk and look for sources that are non-pasteurized, non-homogenized. Homogenization breaks the fat molecules into really small particles that get into your intestines and blood stream, and it's very unhealthy. Do you remember when cream used to rise to the top in the good old days? Well, we don't have that anymore.

- Buy organic local (not long distance) at every opportunity. Grow your own when in doubt. Look for co-ops and CSAs. They are springing up all over the country for meat, chicken, pork, vegetables, fruit, and almost anything you can name. Healthy foods are not that difficult to obtain.

Once more, healthy eating is not that difficult. You won't have trouble falling off and then going back to healthy eating. It's a lifestyle change. It's not a hard one, but you do have to change. I know in the beginning you may long for macaroni and cheese. You may be addicted to soft drinks. Once you do this for a length of time, you will not have that desire; it will go away. You'll feel better. Remember, sugar is more addictive than cocaine.

Remember the promises from the beginning of this book: you want to feel better, look better and take pride in what you do. I was fat. I had trouble bending over because when I did, everything got squashed and I couldn't breathe. It put pressure on my lungs. My joints were bad. I'm doing better. I feel good, and you can too, if you learn the healthy eating secrets revealed in *Dr. Bob's Eat Healthy, Look Better, Live Longer.*

Remember, I'm revealing what the big corporations don't want you to know!

# Questions?

**If you have questions, please contact me at drbobcowblog@gmail.com.**

# References

www.wealthyhealthywise.net
www.drbobthehealthbuilder.com (coming soon)
www.drbobthehealthbuilder.podomatic.com
www.pardonyourhangover.com
www.bardsfarm.com (coming soon)

**White bread; Cereal for breakfast**

> Sally Fallon heads the Weston A. Price Foundation (www.westonaprice.org) and has tapes and other wonderful information available.

**Milk for calcium**

> Fallon www.westonaprice.org *Nourishing Traditions*
> www.realmilk.com

**Juice**

Fallon www.westonaprice.org

**Artificial Sweeteners**

H.J. Roberts, MD, *Aspartame: Is It Safe?* (Charles Press Pubs, Sept. 1992) and Dr Mercola, DO, *Sweet Deception*

**Excitotoxins**

Russell L. Blaylock, MD, *Excitotoxins: The Taste That Kills* (Health Press, Dec. 1996)

**Fats**

Fallon

Dr. Arden Andersen, *Real Medicine, Real Health* (Acres USA, Sept. 2004)

**Vegetable Oils**

Fallon www.westonaprice.org

Andersen www.acresusa.com

**AHA Diet**

Andersen

**Companies/Government and obesity**

Sally Fallon www.westonaprice.org

Dr Arden Andersen, DO

Sherry A. Rogers, MD, books available at www.prestigepublishing.com ,

Dr Doris Rapp, MD at www.drrapp.com

### Chemicals in farming
www.acresusa.com

### Need to detoxify
Dr Arden Andersen, PhD, DO

www.acresusa.com

Dr. H.R. Roberts, MD

Dr. Russell Blaylock, MD

Dr. Rogers, MD *Detoxify or Die* (Prestige Publishing, Dec. 2002)

### Trace Minerals
www.drbobthehealthbuilder.com

(coming soon)

Andersen

Rogers

Marc Rose, MD and Michael Rose, MD, *Save Your Sight* (Warner Books, Aug. 1998)

www.acresusa.com *Minerals for the Genetic Code* by Charles Walters

### Fish Oils
"Inflammation - The Secret Killer" *Time* (February 23, 2004)

### My doctor tells me to eat lots of fish
Rogers  www.prestigepublishing.com

**Butter is bad for me, right?**

  Andersen

  Fallon www.westonaprice.org is best source

  Rogers

**Five Worst Foods**

  Dr. Joseph Mercola

  www.mercola.com

**Genetically Modified Organisms**

  Jeffery M. Smith, *Seeds of Deception* (Yes!

  Books, Sept. 2003) Also, see

  www.seedsofdeception.com

**Herbicides and Pesticides**

  www.acresusa.com

  Andersen

  Rogers

**Fertilizers (all about toxic fertilizers)**

  Patty Martin, Quincy, WA. Her story is told in the

  book *Fateful Harvest* by Duff Wilson (Harper

  Paperbacks, Oct. 2002). She was the first

  person that I interviewed on my radio show.

**What about salt?**

  Redmond Real Salt, Redmond, UT

  www.redmondminerals.com

**Healthy cheese**

There isn't a lot of healthy cheese produced in the US, but this company in a very small town in eastern Ohio sells cheese made by the Amish. The Amish produce some of the best cheese you will ever eat. Their Swiss is "to die for." Their cheddars (white and yellow) are outstanding. They also make cheddar, bacon, mild horse radish that is beyond anything you will ever find in a store. This company also carries a unique meat product called "Trail Bologna." This is made with quality meats (not the cow's udder and other less desirable leftover parts) and seasoned just right. Trail Bologna and Swiss cheese is a great healthy snack. They are not very high tech, no website, but they ship UPS to any place in the US. In the winter, you can have it shipped on Monday and received on Thursday. In warmer weather you can have it shipped same day UPS.

Ables cheese, Sardis, Ohio 800 355 5313

**Filtered clean water and FIR sauna**
www.hightechhealth.com
High Tech Health
Are you going the be the filter that takes chemicals out of the water, or are you going to buy a filter that cleans the water for you? This is the best filter I have found, and my wife and I use it every day to drink and to cook our food.

**Healthy meat**

I suggest you buy local grass-fed meat when you can (www.eatwild.com), but that is not always possible. US Wellness Meats are outstanding and their shipping will guarantee freshness. The information in their e-mails is valuable.

US Wellness Meats (www.uswellnessmeats.com).

Pardon™ Hangover Helper – When You Absolutely Have Too Function Tomorrow (www.pardonyourhangover.com). This humate product can lower blood alcohol levels (when you are a little queasy). It will also prevent headaches and sickness the next day.

Humates FP has lowered blood sugar, lowered high blood pressure, prevented the pain and other symptoms of herpes (by restoring the immune system), changed positive pap smears to negative (in 60 to 90 days in 82 % of women in one study taking this supplement), and prevented anxiety attacks from people trying to get off SSRI mind altering legal drugs. There are other people with chronic viral health conditions that have been in remission for several years. My sister suffers from MS and her symptoms are less when she takes 50 mg per day.

To Your Good Health,
Dr. Robert D. Bard, OD, FAAO, ONS
(Dr. Bob the Health Builder)

(214) 615-6505, ext. 1748
PO Box 914
Whitesboro, TX 76273-0884
www.wealthyhealthywise.net
www.drbobthehealthbuilder.com (coming soon)
www.drbobthehealthbuilder.podomatic.com
www.pardonyourhangover.com
www.bardsfarm.com (coming soon)
www.eathealthyu.com

**Final thought**: I am increasingly convinced that sugar and high fructose corn syrup may be the worst things in our diets. Sugars cause Type II diabetes and make many cancers worse. Check out *Sugar Shock!* by Connie Bennett, C.H.H.C.

Watch for my new book
www.organicfarmingandgardeningtips.com
One hundred years ago there was no diabetes, few heart attacks and cancer was only three percent of total deaths. I have put together a recipe book of foods that people ate one hundred years ago when chronic disease was unheard of in the US. You will have an opportunity to eat healthy. This can down loaded FREE plus S and H at www.eathealthyU.com.